Table Of Contents

Chapter 1: Introduction to Ethical AI in Care Homes

The Need for Change in Residential Care

The residential care sector is at a crossroads, facing increasing scrutiny regarding the quality of care provided to the elderly and vulnerable populations. Traditional models of care often prioritize profit over patient well-being, leading to a proliferation of facilities that may cut corners by employing inadequately trained staff. This approach not only jeopardizes the dignity and safety of residents but also undermines the overall mission of care homes, which should be to foster a nurturing and supportive environment. As the demand for quality elder care continues to rise, it becomes essential to reassess and redefine the operational paradigms within the sector.

Generative Artificial Intelligence Gen AI Improving the care of elderly and vulnerable people in care homes. Unfortunately, too common in current society are private care homes owners who are ruthless, focused on profiteering and so self-centred they don't see how providing poor or lo quality support to those who pay to be in their care homes effects not just the individual but their families, loved ones and has a cost to the NHS, Much of the care is paid by UK Taxpayers but also some that is paid for by the individuals in care by selling their homes and assets. A hard journey if you spent your life earning working hard to ern those assets, but the private care homeowners only care about their profit, their own enjoyment often going on holidays and buying holiday homes in Dubai thoughtless about the care they are supposed to provide. Its much worse then that , where elderly with no support give up their homes, these ruthless private care home owners take over their homes at a discounted price to give their 20 year old children homes in posh areas like Hampton , London UK . Setting a bad example to their own children on how to profit from others hardship. Its an abuse of the system that can't be ignored, its not sustainable in the future with a growing ageing population. Gen AI is changing that equation more in favour of the elderly and those that need care in later years. Some reputable large companies with care homes have allready adopted the technology while rogue monetary focus private care owners still look at ways to avoid accountability. The challenges associated with an ageing society have been well documented. By 2040, 64% of the UK's population will be over 65 years old, and this means people are living with ailments for longer, emphasising the growing need for services that care for the demands of an ageing population. The elderly care sector, which incorporates care homes, assisted living, specialist care homes, and in-home care, has been a mixed bag. Ruthless private care homeowners still focus on profit while ethical larger companies have been exploring ways to improve standard of care for residents without increasing the financial burden. If someone you love needs a care home these are things to consider and ask are they adopting HAI and how can they show you? . Energy inflation and wage rises have pushed up costs significantly, some ruthless private care homes have attempted to secure their profits by employing unqualified cheap work force, while more ethical care homes are exploring ways to mitigate rises without passing on cost increases to residents' fees or compromising on standards. Generative Artificial intelligence (Gen AI) is here to help. It is allready being adopted across major industries, so it is understandable that healthcare providers have been keen to adopt GEN AI. Reputable Care home providers are already leveraging Gen AI and using the pre-emptive technology to reduce falls, monitor vulnerable residents, detect discomfort and pain in non-verbal residents.

These advancements not only reduce hospital admissions but also improve outcomes for residents. Kuldeepuk Kohli, an advocate of making life better for all utilising Gen AI to reduce financial burden that some can't afford. Kuldeepuk Kohli can help the care sector and care homes see how they can benefit those in their care and still be financially viable using Gen AI . Amongst the options it includes. Wearable technology. Care home operators have already embraced technology to improve residents' care through digital innovations. Technologies such as robotics, interactive programmes, and digital care records, bringing a multitude of benefits to care, residents, and their families. One of the most recent innovations include wearable devices which have been trialled in care homes across the UK to enhance independence and autonomy, while staying connected. Lightweight devices are designed to distinguish from residents participating in day-to-day activities and residents who have been hurt from falls. Wearable technology can also set medication reminders and records when and which medication has been taken, reducing the possibility of missing doses or overmedicating, increasing positive health outcomes for residents. Kuldeepuk Kohli can help with over two decades experience in the field.

The integration of generative artificial intelligence (Gen AI) offers a transformative opportunity to pivot from an outdated focus on financial gains towards a model centered on ethical care. AI technologies can be employed to streamline administrative tasks, thus reducing overhead costs that can detract from direct care services. By reallocating resources more efficiently, care homes can invest in well-trained staff, ensuring that all personnel are equipped with the skills necessary to provide high-quality care. This shift not only enhances the care experience for residents but also promotes a more sustainable business model for care home operators.

Moreover, ethical AI implementation can lead to personalized care strategies tailored to individual resident needs and preferences. Through data-driven insights, care facilities can create AI-assisted recreational activities that promote engagement and enhance the quality of life for residents. These activities can be customized based on each individual's history, interests, and cognitive abilities, fostering a sense of belonging and purpose. Such tailored experiences are crucial for maintaining mental and emotional well-being, significantly improving residents' overall health outcomes.

The necessity for change is also underscored by the growing demand for transparency and accountability in care home practices. By harnessing AI technologies, facilities can gather and analyze data that inform policy decisions and operational practices. This data-driven approach not only enhances the quality of care but also provides stakeholders, including families and regulatory bodies, with the confidence that their loved ones are receiving the best possible care. With AI, care homes can identify trends, track performance metrics, and implement evidence-based practices that elevate care standards across the board.

In conclusion, the need for change in residential care is pressing and multifaceted. Embracing ethical AI practices can fundamentally reshape the care landscape, moving away from the era of profit-driven facilities towards a future where the well-being of residents takes precedence. Private care home owners, NHS officials, and healthcare providers must collaborate to champion this transformation, ensuring that the care provided is not only efficient but also compassionate and dignified. The potential for improved outcomes through AI is immense, and by committing to these changes, the sector can truly honor its mission to serve the most vulnerable members of our society.

Overview of Generative AI Technologies

Generative AI technologies represent a transformative force in the landscape of care for elderly and vulnerable individuals residing in care homes. These technologies, which include advanced machine learning algorithms capable of creating text, images, and even music, can be harnessed to enhance the quality of care provided in residential facilities. By leveraging generative AI, care providers can create personalized experiences that cater to the unique preferences and needs of each resident, ultimately fostering a more engaging and supportive environment. This shift not only emphasizes the importance of individualized care but also helps to move away from the traditional model of care that often prioritizes profit over quality.

One of the most significant benefits of generative AI in care homes is its potential to assist in the management of resources efficiently. Through data analysis and predictive modeling, AI can help care home owners optimize staffing levels, ensuring that trained professionals are allocated where they are needed most. This not only reduces operational costs but also enhances the quality of care, as residents receive attention from competent staff members rather than untrained individuals. Implementing AI-driven resource management strategies can lead to a more sustainable model for care homes, aligning financial viability with the ethical obligation to provide high-quality services.

Generative AI can also play a pivotal role in creating tailored recreational activities for residents. By analyzing individual preferences and social interactions, AI technologies can generate activity recommendations that resonate with specific residents, promoting engagement and mental well-being. This personalized approach to recreational programming not only enriches the lives of residents but also fosters a sense of community within care homes. By shifting focus from generic activities to those that genuinely interest residents, care homes can enhance the overall experience for elderly individuals, contributing to their happiness and satisfaction.

Moreover, the implementation of ethical AI practices is crucial in the context of care homes. As generative AI technologies become more integrated into daily operations, it is essential to establish guidelines that prioritize the dignity and privacy of residents. Care home providers must be vigilant in ensuring that AI systems are designed and deployed with transparency and accountability. This includes safeguarding sensitive data and ensuring that the use of AI does not compromise the ethical standards of care. By prioritizing ethical AI implementation, care homes can build trust with residents and their families, demonstrating a commitment to responsible and compassionate care.

Finally, generative AI enables care homes to harness data-driven insights that can inform policy and practice improvements. By analyzing patterns in resident behavior, feedback, and health outcomes, AI can provide valuable insights that help care providers make informed decisions. This data-centric approach not only enhances the quality of care but also supports continuous improvement within care home environments. As the sector evolves, the integration of generative AI technologies will be essential in shaping future policies that prioritize the well-being of elderly and vulnerable populations, ultimately leading to a reformed care landscape that is both ethical and efficient.

The Role of Ethics in AI Implementation

The integration of artificial intelligence (AI) into residential care facilities presents unique ethical challenges and opportunities, particularly in the context of elderly and vulnerable populations. As private care home owners, NHS representatives, and healthcare professionals explore the implementation of AI technologies, it is crucial to prioritize ethical considerations to ensure that these innovations serve the best interests of residents. Ethical AI practices not only enhance the quality of care but also mitigate the risks associated with data privacy, consent, and potential biases in AI algorithms. By establishing a framework grounded in ethical principles, care homes can foster an environment where technology complements compassionate care.

One of the fundamental aspects of ethical AI implementation in care homes is the protection of residents' rights and dignity. In an era where data is a valuable commodity, ensuring informed consent becomes paramount. Residents and their families must be made fully aware of how their data will be utilized and the implications of AI technologies on their care. This includes being transparent about the capabilities and limitations of AI tools. By prioritizing informed consent and maintaining open lines of communication, care homes can build trust with residents and their families, thereby enhancing the overall care experience.

Moreover, the deployment of AI in care environments should aim to reduce inequities rather than exacerbate them. AI algorithms can inadvertently perpetuate biases if not carefully designed and monitored. It is essential for care home operators to collaborate with experts in AI ethics to ensure that the systems they implement are fair and unbiased. This involves regularly auditing AI tools for discriminatory outcomes and making necessary adjustments to the algorithms. By adopting a proactive approach to bias detection and mitigation, care homes can guarantee that all residents receive equitable treatment and care.

AI also offers opportunities to improve operational efficiency, ultimately reducing care costs without compromising quality. Ethical AI practices promote resource management that aligns with the core mission of care homes: to provide compassionate and individualized care. By utilizing AI for tasks such as scheduling, resource allocation, and predictive analytics, facilities can optimize their operations. This efficiency allows for better staff training and retention, as well as the ability to allocate more resources directly to resident care. Consequently, care homes can transition away from profit-driven models and invest in training qualified staff, fostering a culture of care that prioritizes the well-being of residents.

Lastly, AI can enhance recreational activities tailored to individual preferences, contributing to an improved quality of life for residents. Ethical AI practices encourage the development of systems that respect personal preferences and promote autonomy. By leveraging data-driven insights, care homes can create personalized activity plans that engage residents and encourage social interaction. This not only enriches the residents' daily lives but also supports their mental and emotional well-being. As care homes embrace AI technologies, it is imperative to remain committed to ethical standards that prioritize the needs and preferences of those they serve, ultimately transforming the landscape of elderly care for the better.

Chapter 2: Understanding Generative AI

What is Generative AI?

Generative AI, a subset of artificial intelligence, refers to systems that can create new content and insights based on existing data. Unlike traditional AI, which primarily analyzes and processes information, generative AI goes a step further by producing innovative outputs such as text, images, and even music. This capability can be particularly transformative in the context of elderly care within residential facilities. By leveraging generative AI, care homes can develop personalized experiences that cater to the unique preferences and needs of each resident, thereby enhancing their quality of life.

In the realm of care for elderly and vulnerable individuals, generative AI can take on various roles, from facilitating communication to creating tailored recreational activities. For instance, AI-generated content can provide personalized storytelling or reminiscence therapy, tapping into the rich histories of residents to foster engagement and connection. This not only stimulates cognitive function but also combats feelings of loneliness and isolation, which are prevalent in care home environments. By focusing on individualized care through generative AI, facilities can shift their approach from a one-size-fits-all model to a more nuanced and compassionate framework.

Moreover, the implementation of generative AI can address the pressing issue of staffing quality in private care homes. Many facilities struggle with employing adequately trained staff, often leading to inadequate care. Generative AI can assist in training existing staff by providing them with simulated scenarios and best practices in handling various resident needs. This technology can also help in the recruitment process by streamlining candidate assessments and ensuring that only qualified individuals are selected for caregiving roles, thereby elevating the overall standard of care.

Cost management is another significant advantage of generative AI in residential care settings. By automating routine administrative tasks and optimizing resource allocation, care homes can reduce operational costs while maintaining high-quality care. Generative AI can analyze data patterns to predict resource needs, ensuring that staff are deployed effectively and that supplies are managed efficiently. This not only leads to better financial health for care facilities but also allows for more funds to be allocated towards direct resident care and innovative programming.

Finally, the integration of generative AI offers valuable data-driven insights that can inform care home policies and practices. By analyzing trends in resident behavior, preferences, and outcomes, facility managers can make informed decisions that enhance operational effectiveness and resident satisfaction. These insights can drive continuous improvement in care delivery, fostering an environment that prioritizes the well-being of residents. As generative AI continues to evolve, its potential to reshape the landscape of elderly care by promoting ethical practices and improving quality of life becomes increasingly apparent.

Applications of Generative AI in Elderly Care

The integration of generative AI in elderly care holds transformative potential, offering innovative solutions that enhance the quality of life for residents in care homes. By harnessing AI technologies, care facilities can move beyond traditional methods, which often prioritize profit over patient well-being. Generative AI can facilitate personalized care plans that cater to the unique needs of each resident, ensuring that their physical, emotional, and social requirements are met. This shift not only improves resident satisfaction but also fosters a more humane approach to elderly care, moving away from the era of undertrained staff and profit-driven motives.

One of the most impactful applications of generative AI is its ability to optimize resource management within care homes. By analyzing data on resident needs, staffing levels, and operational costs, AI can provide insights that help administrators allocate resources more efficiently. This not only reduces costs but also ensures that staff are deployed where they are most needed. Consequently, residents benefit from better care, as facilities can maintain appropriate staffing levels and improve overall service without compromising on quality. Such efficiency is particularly vital in an industry often criticized for its financial priorities over genuine care.

Generative AI also plays a crucial role in enhancing recreational activities tailored to individual preferences. By analyzing data about residents' interests, past activities, and social interactions, AI can suggest personalized recreational programs that engage residents and promote socialization. This tailored approach not only enriches the lives of elderly individuals but also encourages meaningful interactions among residents, fostering a sense of community within care homes. These engagements can significantly improve mental health outcomes, reducing feelings of isolation and depression, which are prevalent among the elderly.

Moreover, the ethical implementation of AI in care settings is paramount. Care home owners and managers must prioritize transparency and fairness when integrating AI technologies. This involves ensuring that AI systems are designed with input from care staff, residents, and their families, fostering trust in these new tools. Ethical AI practices can help mitigate biases that may arise in data-driven decision-making, ensuring that all residents receive equitable care. The focus should be on enhancing human oversight rather than replacing it, ensuring that AI serves as a supportive tool for trained professionals rather than a substitute.

Finally, generative AI can provide data-driven insights that inform care home policies and practices. By analyzing patterns in resident health outcomes and service utilization, AI can highlight areas for improvement, guiding leadership in making evidence-based decisions. This capability enables care homes to adapt their practices to better meet the evolving needs of their residents, ultimately leading to improved health outcomes and higher standards of care. As the sector evolves, embracing these technologies responsibly can help end the cycle of neglect and profit-driven motives, paving the way for a more compassionate and effective approach to elderly care.

Challenges and Misconceptions Surrounding AI

The integration of artificial intelligence in care homes presents numerous challenges and misconceptions that must be addressed to fully realize its potential. One significant challenge is the resistance to change among staff and management. Many care home owners are accustomed to traditional methods of care delivery and may view AI as a threat to their current operations or as a complicated addition to their existing systems. This apprehension can lead to a reluctance to adopt AI technologies, even when these tools can enhance care quality and efficiency. Overcoming this resistance requires comprehensive training and a clear communication strategy to highlight the benefits of AI, such as improved patient outcomes and reduced workloads.

Another prevalent misconception is that AI will replace human caregivers rather than augment their capabilities. In reality, AI is designed to support, not supplant, the invaluable human touch that is essential in elderly care. For instance, AI can assist in routine tasks, such as medication management and appointment scheduling, allowing caregivers to devote more time to interpersonal interactions with residents. By emphasizing the role of AI as a complementary resource, care homes can alleviate fears regarding job security and demonstrate how these technologies can improve both care efficiency and staff satisfaction.

Data privacy and security concerns also pose challenges in the implementation of AI in care settings. With the collection of sensitive personal information, care home owners must navigate complex regulations to ensure compliance while protecting residents' privacy. Misunderstandings about data usage can lead to distrust among staff and residents. It is crucial for care home administrators to establish transparent data practices, communicate the measures taken to protect privacy, and involve residents in discussions about how their data will be utilized. Building trust in data management practices is essential for successful AI integration.

Additionally, the potential for biased algorithms is a challenge that cannot be overlooked. AI systems are only as good as the data they are trained on, and if that data reflects existing biases, it can perpetuate inequality in care delivery. Care home owners must be vigilant in selecting AI tools that prioritize fairness and inclusivity. This involves actively seeking out AI solutions that have been tested for bias and ensuring ongoing monitoring of their performance in diverse populations. By prioritizing ethical AI practices, care homes can foster a more equitable environment for all residents.

Lastly, the expectation that AI will lead to immediate cost savings can lead to disappointment if not managed realistically. While AI can contribute to reduced operational costs in the long run, the initial investment in technology, training, and infrastructure can be substantial. Care home owners might misconceive AI as a quick fix for financial issues without understanding the necessity of a thoughtful implementation strategy. A successful transition to AI requires careful planning, continuous evaluation, and openness to adapt strategies based on ongoing feedback. By addressing these challenges and misconceptions, care homes can better navigate the complexities of AI integration and enhance the overall quality of care for elderly and vulnerable populations.

Chapter 3: Transitioning from Profit-Driven Care to Ethical Practices

The Impact of Profit Motive on Care Quality

The profit motive in residential care facilities significantly influences the quality of care provided to elderly and vulnerable individuals. In a landscape increasingly driven by financial considerations, the prioritization of profitability can overshadow the fundamental mission of care homes: to provide compassionate and high-quality care. This focus on financial gain often leads to the employment of untrained staff, inadequate resources, and a lack of personalized attention for residents. The implications of these practices are severe, as they can compromise the well-being of those who are most in need of support and care.

The integration of Generative Artificial Intelligence (Gen AI) presents a transformative opportunity to address the shortcomings associated with profit-driven models. By leveraging AI technologies, care facilities can enhance operational efficiencies, thereby reducing costs without sacrificing care quality. For instance, AI can optimize staffing patterns, ensuring that trained professionals are available when and where they are needed most, thus enhancing the overall standard of care.

This shift from a purely profit-driven approach to one that is informed by data and technology can lead to improved outcomes for residents while maintaining financial viability for care providers.

Ethical AI implementation in care environments is critical to ensuring that the focus remains on enhancing care quality rather than merely reducing costs. By adopting ethical guidelines, care homes can use AI to support decision-making processes that prioritize resident well-being. This can involve developing systems that monitor resident health data in real-time, allowing for timely interventions and personalized care plans. Moreover, ethical AI practices can facilitate a culture of transparency and accountability, where care homes are encouraged to prioritize the needs of their residents over financial gain.

AI-assisted recreational activities tailored to individual preferences also represent a significant advancement in the quality of care. By utilizing AI to analyze personal interests and past activities, care facilities can create engaging and meaningful experiences for residents. This personalized approach not only enhances the quality of life for individuals but also fosters a sense of community and belonging within care homes. Engaging residents in activities that resonate with their personal histories can lead to improved mental health outcomes and overall satisfaction with care services.

Data-driven insights are invaluable for improving care home policies and practices, enabling leaders to make informed decisions that enhance care quality. By analyzing patterns and outcomes, care homes can identify areas needing improvement and implement evidence-based strategies to enhance service delivery. This approach can shift the narrative away from a profit-centric model to one that values care quality and resident satisfaction. Ultimately, the thoughtful integration of AI and ethical practices can help redefine the standards of care in residential facilities, ensuring that the needs of elderly and vulnerable individuals are at the forefront of care delivery.

Case Studies of Ethical Practices in Care Homes

Case studies of ethical practices in care homes illustrate the transformative potential of generative artificial intelligence in enhancing the quality of care for the elderly and vulnerable populations. One notable example is the implementation of AI-driven care management systems in a private care home in the UK. This facility integrated AI technology to assess the needs of residents, allowing staff to personalize care plans based on individual preferences and health requirements. By doing so, the care home not only improved the overall well-being of its residents but also fostered a culture of respect and dignity, moving away from a profit-driven model to one centered on compassionate care.

Another significant case study involves the use of AI-assisted recreational activities tailored to residents' interests. A care home in Canada adopted a generative AI platform that analyzes resident data to recommend personalized activities. This approach enabled staff to curate engaging experiences that resonated with each individual, promoting social interaction and mental stimulation. The success of this initiative highlighted the importance of understanding residents as unique individuals rather than treating them as mere numbers, thereby enhancing their quality of life and encouraging a sense of community within the facility.

In addition to improving resident engagement, ethical AI implementation also plays a critical role in resource management. A care home in Australia utilized AI algorithms to optimize staffing schedules based on the fluctuating needs of residents. By analyzing patterns in care demands, the facility was able to allocate resources more effectively, ensuring that trained staff were available during peak times while also reducing operational costs. This strategic use of AI not only ensured high-quality care but also demonstrated a commitment to ethical practices by prioritizing the well-being of residents over financial gain.

Data-driven insights gained through AI can also inform care home policies and practices. A study conducted in a large care facility in the US showcased how AI analytics were employed to identify trends in resident health outcomes. By leveraging this data, management was able to implement evidence-based improvements in care delivery, ensuring that policies were aligned with the actual needs of residents. This proactive approach reinforced the importance of using technology ethically and responsibly to enhance care standards and foster a supportive environment.

These case studies collectively illustrate the potential for generative AI to revolutionize care practices in residential facilities. By prioritizing ethical considerations and focusing on the individual needs of residents, care homes can transition from traditional, profit-centric models to ones that emphasize dignity, respect, and quality of life. As the sector moves forward, embracing ethical AI practices will be crucial in shaping a future where vulnerable populations receive the compassionate care they deserve.

Strategies for Shifting Focus to Quality Care

The shift towards quality care in residential facilities is essential for enhancing the well-being of elderly and vulnerable individuals. Private care home owners and healthcare professionals must recognize that prioritizing quality over profit is not only an ethical obligation but also a strategic necessity in today's competitive environment. One effective strategy is to integrate generative artificial intelligence (Gen AI) technologies that facilitate personalized care plans. By leveraging data on individual preferences, health conditions, and social needs, care homes can craft tailored experiences that significantly enhance residents' quality of life. This approach reduces reliance on a one-size-fits-all model, fostering an environment that respects the uniqueness of each resident.

Training staff to utilize AI tools effectively is another critical component in the pursuit of quality care. Implementing ethical AI practices requires a well-trained workforce that understands how to interpret data-driven insights and apply them in real-world scenarios. Care homes should invest in comprehensive training programs that focus on both technical skills and empathetic caregiving. This dual focus ensures that staff members not only understand the technology but also how to engage meaningfully with residents, thus creating a supportive atmosphere that prioritizes emotional and physical well-being.

In addition to improving staff capabilities, efficient AI resource management can contribute to reducing care costs while enhancing service quality. By automating routine administrative tasks, care homes can free up valuable time for caregivers to focus on direct patient interactions. AI can also streamline scheduling, medication management, and reporting, allowing for more effective allocation of resources. These efficiencies are crucial for maintaining high standards of care without compromising financial stability, ultimately benefiting both residents and care home owners.

AI-assisted recreational activities tailored to individual preferences can further enrich the lives of residents. By analyzing data on interests and past activities, care homes can design programs that engage residents in meaningful ways. Whether through virtual reality experiences, personalized music playlists, or tailored exercise programs, these activities not only promote physical health but also foster social connections and emotional well-being. Creating an environment where residents can thrive socially and emotionally is a hallmark of quality care that distinguishes ethical care homes from those focused solely on profit.

Finally, data-driven insights can play a vital role in improving care home policies and practices. Regularly analyzing feedback and outcomes allows care homes to adjust their strategies in real time, ensuring that they remain aligned with the needs of their residents. This proactive approach helps in identifying areas for improvement, facilitating a continuous cycle of enhancement in care delivery. By fostering a culture of accountability and responsiveness, care homes can genuinely commit to the principle of quality care, positioning themselves as leaders in the ethical implementation of AI in the healthcare landscape.

Chapter 4: Ethical AI Implementation in Care Home Environments

Principles of Ethical AI in Healthcare

The integration of ethical AI in healthcare, particularly within residential facilities, is critical for ensuring that advancements in technology align with the values of compassion, respect, and dignity for elderly and vulnerable populations. Ethical AI principles serve as a framework that guides the development and deployment of artificial intelligence tools in care settings, promoting not only efficiency but also the well-being of residents. Key principles include transparency, accountability, fairness, and beneficence, which collectively aim to create a supportive environment where technology enhances rather than compromises the quality of care.

Transparency is essential in the implementation of AI systems within care homes. Stakeholders, including care home owners, staff, and residents, must have a clear understanding of how AI technologies operate and make decisions. This involves providing accessible information about the algorithms used, data sources, and potential biases. By fostering an open dialogue about AI functionalities, care homes can build trust with residents and their families, alleviating concerns about privacy and the quality of care. Such transparency not only empowers caregivers to utilize AI effectively but also enables residents to feel more secure in their care environment.

Accountability is another cornerstone of ethical AI in healthcare. Care home owners and operators must establish clear lines of responsibility for AI-driven decisions, ensuring that human oversight is integral to the care process. This means that while AI can assist in tasks such as personalized care recommendations or resource management, the ultimate responsibility for care outcomes rests with trained staff. Implementing robust monitoring systems that track AI performance and its impact on resident care can help identify issues and facilitate continuous improvement. This accountability promotes a culture of safety and reliability in care practices, essential for maintaining high standards in elderly care.

Fairness in AI applications is crucial to avoid discrimination and biases that could adversely affect vulnerable populations. Care home operators must ensure that AI systems are designed to be inclusive and representative of the diverse backgrounds of their residents. This involves using diverse training datasets, regularly assessing AI outputs for fairness, and engaging with residents to understand their unique needs and preferences. By prioritizing fairness, care homes can create a more equitable environment where every resident receives personalized support that respects their individuality and dignity.

Finally, the principle of beneficence emphasizes the importance of using AI to enhance the well-being of residents. Care homes can leverage AI technologies to develop tailored recreational activities that cater to the interests and capabilities of individual residents, promoting social engagement and mental health. Additionally, data-driven insights can inform care home policies and practices, allowing for more efficient resource management and improved care delivery. By aligning AI initiatives with the overarching goal of enhancing resident quality of life, care homes can transition away from profit-driven models towards a more compassionate approach that prioritizes the needs and rights of those they serve.

Building Trust Between AI and Care Staff

Building trust between AI and care staff is essential for the successful integration of artificial intelligence into residential care facilities. This trust is not merely a product of technological efficiency; it also hinges on the human element of care. Care staff must feel confident that AI tools can enhance their work without undermining their professional judgment or the emotional connections they cultivate with residents. To establish this trust, organizations should prioritize transparency in AI operations and decision-making processes. By clearly communicating how AI systems function and how they can support staff in their daily tasks, care homes can foster a collaborative environment where technology is viewed as an ally rather than a competitor.

Training is a critical component in building this trust. Care staff must be equipped with the skills to use AI effectively, ensuring they understand the technology's capabilities and limitations. Training programs should not only focus on the technical aspects of AI but also emphasize its role in enhancing care quality. When staff members see the positive outcomes resulting from AI-assisted processes, such as improved resident engagement or streamlined administrative tasks, their confidence in these tools will grow. This confidence is vital for encouraging staff to adopt AI solutions enthusiastically rather than reluctantly, thus maximizing their potential benefits.

Another essential factor in building trust is involving care staff in the AI implementation process. By soliciting their input and feedback at various stages, organizations can create a sense of ownership among the staff. When care workers feel that their insights are valued, they are more likely to support the introduction of AI technologies. This participatory approach can also lead to the development of AI systems that are better tailored to the specific needs of residents and staff alike. Furthermore, it fosters a culture of collaboration, where technology and human care work in tandem to deliver the highest standards of service.

Ethical considerations play a crucial role in establishing trust between AI and care staff. Care homes must ensure that AI is implemented in a manner that respects the dignity and privacy of residents. This includes safeguarding sensitive data and ensuring that AI-generated insights are utilized responsibly. When care staff observe that ethical standards are upheld in AI usage, their trust in the technology will deepen. Organizations should also create channels for staff to voice concerns regarding ethical dilemmas posed by AI, ensuring that there is a mechanism to address any issues that arise.

Ultimately, the relationship between AI and care staff should be viewed as a partnership aimed at improving the overall quality of care. By prioritizing transparency, comprehensive training, staff involvement, and ethical practices, care homes can cultivate an environment where AI is embraced, not feared. This partnership not only enhances the care experience for residents but also empowers staff, allowing them to focus on what they do best: providing compassionate and personalized care. As the landscape of residential care continues to evolve, fostering this trust will be fundamental to realizing the full potential of AI in transforming the care of elderly and vulnerable individuals.

Training and Support for Care Home Staff

Training and support for care home staff is a critical component in the successful integration of artificial intelligence (AI) within residential facilities. As the landscape of elderly care evolves with the advent of generative AI technologies, it becomes increasingly essential to equip staff with the knowledge and skills necessary to leverage these tools effectively. This training should not only focus on the technical aspects of AI but also emphasize ethical practices that prioritize the well-being of residents. By investing in comprehensive training programs, care home owners can ensure that their staff are not merely users of technology but also advocates for its ethical application in enhancing care.

The importance of a well-structured training curriculum cannot be overstated. It should encompass the fundamentals of AI, its applications in elderly care, and the ethical considerations that arise from its use. Staff members need to understand how AI can assist in areas such as personalized care plans, predictive analytics for health monitoring, and improving communication with residents and their families. By fostering an environment where staff are well-informed about the capabilities and limitations of AI, care homes can help mitigate fears or misconceptions that may arise regarding technology's role in care.

Support systems are equally vital in this process. Care home owners should establish ongoing mentorship and professional development opportunities that allow staff to continuously learn and adapt to new AI advancements. This could include workshops, online courses, and peer support groups where staff can share their experiences and challenges. Furthermore, creating a culture that encourages open dialogue about AI's impact on care practices can enhance staff confidence in utilizing these tools, ultimately leading to better outcomes for residents.

In addition to formal training and support, it is essential to incorporate feedback mechanisms that allow staff to voice their concerns and suggestions regarding AI implementation. These insights can be invaluable for refining care home policies and practices. Engaging staff in the decision-making process not only fosters a sense of ownership but also ensures that the technologies introduced truly meet the needs of both caregivers and residents. Regular assessments of AI tools and their effectiveness in improving care will also help adjust strategies as necessary, ensuring they remain aligned with the overarching goal of enhancing the quality of life for elderly individuals.

Ultimately, a commitment to training and support for care home staff will redefine the standards of care in residential facilities, moving away from a profit-driven model to one that prioritizes compassion and ethical responsibility. By embracing generative AI as a partner in care, rather than a replacement for human interaction, care homes can create environments that empower both staff and residents. This holistic approach will not only improve care delivery but also help restore trust in the care system, demonstrating that the future of elderly care lies in a thoughtful integration of technology and human empathy.

Chapter 5: Reducing Care Costs Through Efficient AI Resource Management

Analyzing Current Cost Structures in Care Homes

Analyzing current cost structures in care homes is essential for understanding how resources are allocated and identifying areas for improvement. Traditional models often prioritize profit over quality, leading to the employment of untrained staff and insufficient care for residents. By examining these cost structures, private care home owners, NHS stakeholders, and health care providers can shift their focus towards ethical practices that enhance the quality of care for elderly and vulnerable individuals. This analysis allows facilities to recognize inefficiencies and implement solutions that not only reduce costs but also improve overall resident satisfaction.

One significant area of cost analysis involves staffing expenses. Care homes frequently face high turnover rates, which can lead to increased recruitment and training costs. The integration of Generative Artificial Intelligence (Gen AI) can streamline workforce management by predicting staffing needs based on resident care requirements. This predictive capability allows care homes to maintain optimal staff levels without overextending budgets. Additionally, AI can assist in identifying candidates with the right skill sets, ensuring that trained professionals are placed in roles where they can make the most impact.

The cost of supplies and equipment is another critical factor in the financial structure of care homes. Many facilities struggle with outdated tools and inefficient inventory management, which can lead to waste and higher operational costs. Ethical AI implementation can assist in optimizing supply chains and inventory management, ensuring that resources are used effectively. By leveraging data-driven insights, care homes can anticipate needs, reduce excess spending, and allocate funds towards enhancing the quality of care rather than unnecessary overhead.

AI-assisted recreational activities tailored to individual preferences represent an innovative approach to enhancing resident engagement while managing costs. Traditional activities are often one-size-fits-all, failing to meet the diverse needs and interests of residents. By utilizing AI to analyze preferences and health conditions, care homes can develop personalized activity programs that not only improve the well-being of residents but also encourage participation and reduce the need for extensive staffing. This tailored approach can lead to better outcomes, demonstrating that thoughtful investment in technology ultimately yields significant returns in care quality.

Lastly, data-driven insights derived from AI can inform care home policies and practices, leading to more effective operational strategies. By analyzing resident data, care homes can identify trends and areas in need of improvement, such as the frequency of falls or medication errors. This proactive approach enables management to implement targeted interventions, thereby reducing costly incidents and enhancing the overall safety and satisfaction of residents. By embracing these analytical practices, care homes can transition away from profit-driven models towards a more compassionate, resident-focused care environment that prioritizes ethical standards and the well-being of those they serve.

AI Solutions for Streamlining Operations

AI solutions are transforming the operational landscape of residential care facilities, presenting opportunities to streamline processes and enhance the quality of care provided to elderly and vulnerable individuals. By integrating Generative Artificial Intelligence (Gen AI) into care home environments, facilities can move away from a profit-driven approach that often leads to inadequate staffing and training. Instead, AI enables a focus on personalized care, ensuring that each resident receives the attention and support they need. This shift not only improves the overall well-being of residents but also fosters a more ethical approach to caregiving.

One of the most significant advantages of AI in care homes is its ability to optimize resource management. AI algorithms can analyze data related to staffing patterns, resident needs, and operational costs, allowing care home owners to allocate resources more effectively. This data-driven approach leads to reduced care costs while ensuring that staffing levels are appropriate for the needs of each resident. By minimizing waste and maximizing efficiency, care homes can reinvest savings into staff training and development, ultimately enhancing the quality of care.

AI also plays a crucial role in designing and implementing recreational activities that are tailored to the individual preferences of residents. Through the use of AI-driven analytics, care facilities can assess the interests and capabilities of each resident, allowing for the creation of personalized activity programs. These activities not only promote social engagement and mental stimulation but also contribute to the overall happiness and well-being of residents. This personalized approach contrasts sharply with the one-size-fits-all activities often seen in traditional care environments, highlighting the importance of individualized care.

Furthermore, AI technology provides valuable data-driven insights that can inform care home policies and practices. By analyzing trends and outcomes related to resident care, facilities can identify areas for improvement and implement evidence-based strategies. This continuous feedback loop allows care homes to adapt to the changing needs of their residents, ensuring that care practices remain relevant and effective. As a result, care home owners can make informed decisions that enhance operational efficiency and improve resident satisfaction.

In conclusion, the integration of AI solutions into residential care facilities presents a significant opportunity for improving operations and elevating the standard of care. By focusing on ethical AI practices, care home owners can create environments that prioritize the well-being of residents and empower trained staff to deliver high-quality care. This transformation not only benefits the residents but also positions care homes as leaders in the evolving landscape of elder care, paving the way for a more compassionate and effective approach to supporting vulnerable populations.

Long-term Financial Benefits of AI Integration

The integration of artificial intelligence (AI) into residential care facilities is not just a technological advancement; it represents a transformative shift towards more sustainable financial practices. For private care home owners and healthcare providers, the long-term financial benefits of AI integration are substantial. By leveraging AI tools, facilities can optimize operational efficiencies, ultimately reducing overhead costs. For instance, AI-driven scheduling systems can ensure that staffing levels are aligned with actual demand, minimizing unnecessary labor costs while maintaining high standards of care. This strategic management of resources leads to a more financially viable operation without compromising the quality of care provided to residents.

Another significant financial advantage lies in the reduction of care costs through efficient AI resource management. AI systems can analyze various data streams, identifying trends and areas where savings can be made. By automating routine tasks, such as medication management and daily health monitoring, care staff can focus their efforts on more personalized aspects of care, enhancing both resident satisfaction and operational effectiveness. This not only leads to better resource allocation but also helps in preventing costly errors associated with manual processes. Over time, these efficiencies can translate into substantial cost savings, helping to ensure the financial health of care facilities.

Moreover, integrating AI into care homes facilitates the development of tailored recreational activities that resonate with individual resident preferences. By using generative AI to curate personalized experiences, care homes can enhance the well-being of their residents, which is beneficial for both the residents and the facility's bottom line. Engaged residents are generally healthier and more satisfied, leading to reduced turnover rates and lower recruitment costs. Investing in AI-assisted recreational programs can thus yield a dual advantage: improving the quality of life for residents while simultaneously fostering a positive reputation that attracts new clients.

Data-driven insights derived from AI analytics are invaluable for improving care home policies and practices. By continuously monitoring and evaluating resident outcomes, care homes can identify effective strategies and areas needing improvement. This evidence-based approach not only enhances the quality of care but also supports compliance with regulatory standards, potentially reducing the risk of costly penalties. Furthermore, facilities that demonstrate a commitment to high standards of care through data-driven practices are likely to see increased demand from families seeking the best possible environment for their loved ones.

In conclusion, the long-term financial benefits of AI integration in residential care facilities are multifaceted. From operational efficiencies and cost reduction to enhanced resident engagement and data-driven decision-making, AI presents a compelling case for investment in the future of care. By adopting ethical AI practices, care home owners can not only improve their financial stability but also contribute to a more compassionate and effective care system for the elderly and vulnerable populations. This shift away from profit-driven motives towards a model centered on quality care signifies a pivotal moment in the evolution of residential care, ensuring that ethical considerations and financial sustainability go hand in hand.

Chapter 6: AI-Assisted Recreational Activities Tailored to Individual Preferences

Understanding the Importance of Recreation in Elderly Care

Recreation plays a crucial role in the overall well-being of elderly individuals, especially in care home settings. Engaging in recreational activities not only enhances physical health but also significantly contributes to mental and emotional wellness. For private care home owners and healthcare professionals, recognizing the value of recreation is essential in creating environments that foster happiness and satisfaction among residents. As we explore the integration of generative artificial intelligence into elderly care, it becomes evident that AI can help tailor recreational activities to meet the unique needs and preferences of each resident, thereby improving their quality of life.

The benefits of recreational activities extend beyond mere enjoyment; they are vital for maintaining cognitive function and social interaction among the elderly. Activities such as games, arts and crafts, and group outings encourage residents to connect with one another, reducing feelings of loneliness and isolation. For care home operators, implementing structured recreational programs can lead to a more vibrant community atmosphere. By utilizing AI-driven data insights, care homes can design activities that resonate with the interests of their residents, ensuring that participation levels remain high and that activities are meaningful.

Moreover, the ethical implementation of AI in care facilities can streamline the management of recreational resources, reducing costs while enhancing the quality of care. By analyzing data on resident preferences, AI can assist in scheduling and optimizing activities that cater to different ability levels and interests. This efficient resource management helps care homes allocate staff and materials more effectively, allowing trained professionals to focus on delivering high-quality interactions rather than administrative tasks. Consequently, it addresses the critical issue of employing adequately trained staff, moving away from the era of neglect and insufficient care.

AI-assisted recreational activities can also serve as a tool for personalized care. Through continuous learning algorithms, AI can adapt activities based on residents' changing needs or preferences over time. For example, if a resident enjoys painting but shows a decline in fine motor skills, the AI can suggest modified activities that still allow for creative expression without frustration. This tailored approach not only enhances the engagement of residents but also promotes a sense of agency and autonomy, which is vital for their dignity and self-esteem.

Finally, the integration of recreational programming into care home policies requires a paradigm shift in how we view elderly care. By prioritizing recreation as an essential component of health and well-being, care homes can foster a culture that values holistic approaches to care. With the advent of ethical AI practices, the future of elderly care can move toward more compassionate, efficient, and individualized care strategies. This shift not only enhances the lives of residents but also sets a new standard for care home operations, encouraging a more humane and respectful approach to elderly care.

Designing AI Programs for Personalized Activities

Designing AI programs for personalized activities in care homes represents a significant advancement in the quality of care provided to elderly and vulnerable residents. By leveraging generative artificial intelligence, facility operators can create tailored recreational activities that not only engage residents but also promote their overall well-being. These AI-driven programs can assess individual preferences and capabilities, offering a customized experience that traditional methods may overlook. This shift toward personalized care aligns with the ethical considerations that demand a humane approach in residential settings, moving away from profit-driven motives to a focus on genuine resident satisfaction and enrichment.

Effective implementation of AI in care home environments requires careful consideration of both ethical standards and operational efficiency. AI programs should be designed to respect the dignity and autonomy of residents while also addressing their unique needs. By incorporating feedback from caregivers and family members, these systems can ensure that the activities offered resonate with the residents' historical interests and current abilities. This participatory approach not only enhances the effectiveness of the AI systems but also fosters a sense of community and belonging among residents, which is crucial for their emotional health.

Reducing care costs through efficient AI resource management is another critical aspect of designing these programs. By automating routine tasks and optimizing scheduling for activities, care homes can allocate resources more effectively, allowing staff to focus on providing quality care. AI can analyze data to identify trends in resident engagement and resource usage, enabling facilities to make informed decisions about staff allocation and activity planning. This efficiency not only reduces operational costs but also enhances the overall care experience by ensuring that residents receive the attention they need when they need it.

AI-assisted recreational activities can be tailored to individual preferences, ensuring that each resident has the opportunity to participate in meaningful and enjoyable experiences. For instance, AI systems can curate music playlists, suggest art projects, or even organize virtual reality experiences based on the interests of each resident. By providing a diverse range of activities that cater to varying cognitive and physical abilities, care homes can foster an inclusive environment where all residents feel valued and engaged. This personalized approach not only improves the quality of life for residents but also promotes a positive atmosphere within the care home.

Lastly, data-driven insights generated by AI can lead to improved policies and practices within care homes. By analyzing participant engagement and feedback, facilities can refine their activity offerings and develop best practices that align with resident preferences. This continuous improvement cycle allows care homes to adapt to changing needs and ensure that their programs remain relevant and effective. By prioritizing ethical AI practices, care homes can transform their operations, prioritizing the well-being of residents over financial gain and ultimately redefining the standards of care in the industry.

Measuring the Impact of AI on Resident Well-being

Measuring the impact of artificial intelligence (AI) on resident well-being is a complex yet essential endeavor for care home owners and healthcare professionals. The integration of generative AI into residential care settings provides a wealth of opportunities to enhance the quality of life for elderly and vulnerable individuals. By employing AI technologies, care homes can deliver personalized experiences that cater to individual preferences, ultimately fostering a more engaging and fulfilling environment for residents. It is crucial to develop clear metrics to assess how these technologies contribute to resident satisfaction, mental health, and overall quality of life.

One of the primary methods for gauging the impact of AI on well-being is the collection of quantitative data, which includes metrics such as resident engagement levels, frequency of social interactions, and participation in recreational activities. AI can facilitate tailored recreational activities, enhancing the likelihood that residents will participate in activities they find enjoyable. By analyzing patterns in participation and engagement, care home managers can better understand the types of activities that resonate with their residents and adjust programming accordingly. This data-driven approach not only boosts resident satisfaction but also cultivates a sense of community and belonging among individuals who may otherwise feel isolated.

Qualitative assessments, such as resident feedback and caregiver observations, complement quantitative data in measuring AI's impact. Through surveys and interviews, care homes can gather insights into residents' emotional responses to AI-assisted initiatives. For instance, understanding how residents perceive AI-generated music therapy or virtual reality experiences can help care providers fine-tune these offerings to maximize their benefits. Additionally, caregiver observations are invaluable; staff members can provide context about how AI tools influence daily interactions and overall resident mood, leading to more informed decisions on AI implementation.

Furthermore, ethical AI practices play a pivotal role in ensuring that technological advancements genuinely enhance resident well-being. Care home owners must prioritize transparency and consent when deploying AI solutions, ensuring that residents and their families are informed about how data is collected and used. By fostering an environment of trust, facilities can enhance residents' comfort with AI technologies, which in turn can lead to more positive outcomes. Ethical considerations must be woven into the fabric of AI integration, ensuring that the focus remains on improving resident care rather than merely cutting costs or maximizing profits.

Ultimately, measuring the impact of AI on resident well-being is not merely about collecting data; it is about creating a culture of continuous improvement within care homes. By leveraging AI to gather insights and implement necessary adjustments, care facilities can transform the narratives surrounding elderly care. This shift toward ethical AI practices not only elevates the standard of care but also signifies the end of an era marked by inadequate staffing and profit-driven motives. Through thoughtful implementation and assessment of AI technologies, care homes can truly enhance the

lives of their residents, fostering dignity, respect, and well-being for
all.

Chapter 7: Data-Driven Insights for Improving Care Home Policies and Practices

The Role of Data in Enhancing Care Quality

The integration of data into care home operations has emerged as a
pivotal factor in enhancing care quality for elderly and vulnerable
populations. By harnessing the power of data analytics, care home
owners can gain valuable insights into resident needs, preferences,
and health outcomes. This information enables tailored approaches
to care that not only improve the overall well-being of residents but
also foster a more responsive and adaptive care environment.
Through systematic data collection and analysis, care homes can
shift from a one-size-fits-all model to personalized care that respects
the individuality of each resident.

Ethical AI practices play a crucial role in this data-driven approach.
By implementing AI technologies that prioritize ethical
considerations, care homes can ensure that data is used responsibly
and transparently. This not only builds trust among residents and
their families but also aligns with regulatory standards and best
practices in the healthcare industry. AI systems can analyze vast
amounts of data to identify patterns and trends, helping care
providers make informed decisions that enhance care delivery while
protecting resident privacy. The ethical use of data fosters a culture
of accountability and continuous improvement within care facilities.

Moreover, data-driven insights can lead to significant cost reductions
in care home operations. By utilizing AI for resource management,

care homes can optimize staffing levels, reduce waste, and enhance operational efficiency. Predictive analytics can forecast staffing needs based on resident acuity and demand, allowing facilities to employ trained staff more effectively and reduce reliance on untrained personnel. This strategic approach not only lowers operational costs but also elevates the quality of care provided, ensuring that residents receive the attention and expertise they deserve.

AI-assisted recreational activities, tailored to individual preferences, represent another innovative application of data in care homes. By analyzing resident data related to interests, past activities, and social interactions, care homes can create personalized engagement programs that promote mental and emotional well-being. These tailored activities not only improve the quality of life for residents but also encourage community building within the facility. Engaging residents in activities that resonate with their personal histories and preferences fosters a sense of belonging and purpose, which is essential for overall health in elderly populations.

In conclusion, the role of data in enhancing care quality within residential facilities cannot be overstated. By adopting ethical AI practices and leveraging data-driven insights, care homes can transform their operations to prioritize the well-being of residents. This shift not only addresses the historical shortcomings of some care facilities focused solely on profit but also establishes a new standard for care that values compassion, quality, and integrity. As private care home owners, NHS professionals, and elderly care providers embrace these innovations, the future of care can be reimagined to create environments where vulnerable populations thrive.

Utilizing AI for Policy Development

Utilizing AI for policy development in residential care facilities represents a transformative opportunity for private care home owners, NHS administrators, and health care providers. By leveraging generative artificial intelligence, care homes can shift from traditional, profit-driven models towards a more ethical and holistic approach that prioritizes the well-being of elderly and vulnerable residents. AI can assist in formulating policies that enhance care standards, ensuring that trained staff are prioritized over unskilled labor, thus elevating the overall quality of care provided to residents.

One of the key benefits of utilizing AI in policy development is its ability to analyze vast amounts of data to identify trends and areas for improvement. By employing data-driven insights, care home administrators can craft policies that address specific needs within their facilities. This includes evaluating staff training programs, optimizing resource allocation, and ensuring that care practices align with the latest ethical standards. Such informed decision-making is crucial for transitioning away from practices that have historically prioritized profit over quality care.

AI can also support the implementation of ethical guidelines within care home environments. By integrating AI systems that monitor compliance with regulatory standards, care homes can ensure that they are meeting legal and ethical obligations. This technology can track staff qualifications, training progress, and resident satisfaction, providing a comprehensive view of how well the facility adheres to its mission of delivering compassionate care. This proactive approach not only fosters a culture of accountability but also enhances the reputation of care homes committed to ethical practices.

Reducing care costs through efficient AI resource management is another significant advantage. AI can streamline operations by automating administrative tasks, optimizing scheduling, and improving inventory management. By minimizing waste and reallocating resources where they are needed most, care homes can reduce overhead costs while maintaining a high standard of care. This efficiency not only leads to financial savings but also allows for reinvestment in staff training and development, ensuring that caregivers are well-equipped to meet the diverse needs of residents.

Furthermore, AI-assisted recreational activities tailored to individual preferences can enhance the quality of life for residents. By analyzing data on residents' interests and histories, AI can recommend personalized activities that promote engagement and social interaction. This not only improves residents' mental and emotional well-being but also fosters a sense of community within the care home. As policies evolve to incorporate these innovative approaches, the focus will shift towards creating nurturing environments that value the dignity and individuality of each resident, marking a significant departure from the past practices that prioritized profits over people.

Case Studies of Successful Data-Driven Implementations

The implementation of data-driven approaches in residential care has proven transformative, showcasing how technology can enhance the quality of life for elderly and vulnerable individuals. One notable case study is that of a private care home in the UK that integrated a generative artificial intelligence system to personalize care plans based on real-time health data. By utilizing AI algorithms to analyze residents' medical histories, preferences, and daily activities, the facility was able to tailor care strategies that improved both health outcomes and resident satisfaction. This proactive approach not only reduced emergency interventions but also fostered a sense of autonomy among residents, shifting the focus from merely managing health crises to promoting overall well-being.

Another significant example comes from a healthcare provider in Canada that adopted an ethical AI framework to streamline operational efficiencies. By implementing AI-driven resource management tools, the organization reduced staffing costs while ensuring that care standards remained high. These tools analyzed workflows and identified areas where staff could be deployed more effectively. As a result, the facility minimized instances of understaffing during peak hours, which often led to inadequate care. This case highlights the importance of ethical AI implementation, ensuring that technology serves as an enabler rather than a replacement for human care.

In the realm of recreational activities, a care home in Australia utilized AI to create personalized engagement programs. By analyzing resident data, including cognitive abilities and personal interests, the facility developed tailored recreational activities that resonated with each individual. These AI-assisted programs not only improved participation rates among residents but also contributed to enhanced mental health outcomes. This case exemplifies how data-driven insights can be harnessed to create meaningful experiences, demonstrating that technology can enrich the lives of those in care without overshadowing the human touch that is central to caregiving.

A comprehensive study conducted in a network of care homes in the United States focused on policy improvement through data analytics. By collecting and analyzing large datasets on resident outcomes, staff performance, and resource allocation, the organization was able to identify trends that informed policy changes. This data-driven approach led to the implementation of best practices in care delivery and highlighted areas for staff training and development. The organization not only improved care quality but also fostered a culture of continuous learning and adaptation, positioning itself as a leader in ethical AI practices within the sector.

These case studies illustrate the potential of data-driven implementations in transforming care environments. By focusing on ethical AI practices, facilities can enhance care delivery while simultaneously reducing costs and improving resident engagement. The shift towards a more humane and effective model of care is not merely a technological advancement but a necessary evolution in how we approach the needs of the elderly and vulnerable populations in residential settings. As more care homes adopt similar strategies, the industry moves closer to ending the era of profit-driven practices that neglect the fundamental principles of compassionate care.

Chapter 8: Future Trends in AI and Elderly Care

Advances in AI Technology and Their Implications

Advances in artificial intelligence (AI) technology are transforming the landscape of elderly and vulnerable care in residential facilities. Generative AI, in particular, stands out for its potential to enhance the quality of care while addressing longstanding issues associated with profit-driven motives in the care sector. By employing AI-driven tools, care homes can shift their focus from mere financial gains to delivering personalized and compassionate care, ensuring that residents receive the attention and support they need. This transition not only benefits the residents but also fosters a healthier work environment for staff, potentially alleviating the challenges posed by high turnover rates and inadequate training.

Ethical AI implementation is crucial in this context. Care home owners must prioritize the development and deployment of technologies that uphold the dignity and rights of residents. This involves establishing clear guidelines for AI use, ensuring that systems are designed with transparency, accountability, and fairness in mind. By integrating ethical considerations into AI practices, care facilities can avoid the pitfalls of prioritizing profits over people, thereby creating an environment where technology serves to enhance human interaction rather than replace it. This approach can lead to more effective communication and deeper connections between staff and residents, ultimately improving the overall quality of care.

One of the most significant benefits of AI in care homes is the potential for cost reduction through efficient resource management.

AI systems can analyze data related to staffing, inventory, and resident needs, helping administrators make informed decisions that optimize resource allocation. This not only reduces operational costs but also allows care homes to reinvest savings into staff training and development. With a well-trained workforce, facilities can ensure that residents receive high-quality care from knowledgeable professionals who are equipped to meet their specific needs, further enhancing the care experience.

AI-assisted recreational activities tailored to individual preferences represent another exciting advancement in this field. By utilizing AI algorithms that analyze residents' interests and histories, care homes can offer personalized activities that engage and stimulate residents mentally and socially. This tailored approach not only improves the quality of life for individuals but also fosters community among residents, promoting social interaction and reducing feelings of isolation. These advancements in recreational programming can lead to increased satisfaction among residents and their families, making care homes more appealing options for potential clients.

Finally, data-driven insights provided by AI can significantly enhance care home policies and practices. By collecting and analyzing data from various sources, care facilities can identify trends and areas for improvement, enabling proactive adjustments to their operations. This evidence-based approach allows for continuous quality improvement, ensuring that care homes are responsive to the evolving needs of their residents. As AI technology continues to evolve, its potential to revolutionize the care sector becomes increasingly apparent, promising a future where ethical practices and high-quality care are the norm rather than the exception.

Preparing for the Future of Care Homes

Preparing for the future of care homes necessitates a paradigm shift that embraces ethical artificial intelligence as a cornerstone of operations. The integration of generative AI in residential facilities can revolutionize the way care is delivered to elderly and vulnerable individuals. By transitioning from an era where profit margins overshadowed resident welfare to a model focused on compassionate care, private care home owners and healthcare providers can enhance the quality of life for residents. This transformation demands a commitment to training staff in AI technologies and ensuring that ethical practices guide all technological implementations.

Incorporating AI into care home environments offers the potential to significantly reduce operational costs while maintaining or improving care quality. Efficient AI resource management allows facilities to optimize staffing schedules, predict resident needs, and allocate resources more effectively. By employing data-driven insights, care home administrators can identify patterns in resident behaviors and preferences, enabling tailored care plans that enhance individual experiences. This shift not only improves resident satisfaction but also ensures that financial resources are used judiciously, fostering a more sustainable business model.

Moreover, AI-assisted recreational activities can be designed to cater to the unique preferences of each resident, promoting engagement and social interaction. By utilizing generative AI to create personalized activities, care homes can foster an environment where residents feel valued and understood. This approach not only enhances the emotional well-being of residents but also encourages staff to focus on building genuine relationships, thereby reducing the reliance on untrained workers who may not prioritize the emotional and psychological needs of residents.

The ethical implementation of AI in care homes must prioritize transparency, accountability, and inclusivity. It is essential for care home leaders to engage with stakeholders—including residents, families, and healthcare professionals—throughout the AI integration process. This collaboration ensures that the technologies deployed align with the values and expectations of the community served. Furthermore, ongoing training and development for staff will be critical in addressing the ethical implications of AI usage, ensuring that all personnel are equipped to navigate the complexities of technology in a sensitive and responsible manner.

As care homes prepare for this future, they must also consider the regulatory landscape surrounding AI technologies. Adapting to evolving policies, standards, and best practices will be vital in maintaining compliance and safeguarding the interests of residents. By proactively engaging with regulatory bodies and participating in discussions about ethical AI practices, care home owners can lead the charge in establishing a new standard for care that prioritizes both innovation and human dignity. This forward-thinking approach will ultimately contribute to a more compassionate, efficient, and ethically responsible care environment for all.

The Role of Stakeholders in Shaping Future Practices

The involvement of stakeholders in shaping the future practices of care homes is critical for developing an ethical and effective framework for implementing generative artificial intelligence (Gen AI). Stakeholders, including private care home owners, NHS representatives, healthcare professionals, and community organizations, have unique perspectives and contributions that can lead to a collective vision for improving the care of elderly and vulnerable individuals. Engaging these stakeholders in discussions about AI integration ensures that the technology aligns with the needs and values of those it serves, fostering a culture of shared responsibility and ethical oversight.

Private care home owners play a pivotal role in determining the operational practices within their facilities. By embracing ethical AI practices, they can shift away from a profit-centric model that prioritizes financial gain over quality care. The implementation of AI-driven solutions can streamline operations, reduce costs, and improve staff training and retention. Owners who actively engage with technology not only enhance their facilities' reputations but also demonstrate a commitment to ethical standards in elder care, ultimately leading to better outcomes for residents.

Healthcare professionals, including nurses and care staff, are essential stakeholders in the successful integration of AI in care homes. Their frontline experiences provide invaluable insights into the practical challenges and opportunities that AI can address. By involving these professionals in the development and deployment of AI systems, care homes can ensure that the technology enhances their capabilities rather than complicating their workflows. Training programs focused on both AI literacy and ethical practices can empower staff, allowing them to leverage technology effectively while maintaining the human touch that is vital in caregiving.

Community organizations and advocacy groups also play a significant role in shaping future practices within care homes. Their advocacy for the rights and needs of elderly residents can guide the ethical implementation of AI technologies. By fostering partnerships with these organizations, care homes can gain access to resources and support networks that promote best practices in resident care. Furthermore, community input can help ensure that AI applications are sensitive to the cultural and individual preferences of residents, making care more personalized and effective.

Lastly, data-driven insights generated from AI systems can inform care home policies and practices, leading to continuous improvement. Stakeholders must collaborate to establish frameworks that prioritize data privacy and ethical considerations while harnessing the potential of AI analytics. By utilizing these insights, care homes can better understand resident needs, optimize resource allocation, and enhance overall care quality. In this way, the collective involvement of stakeholders not only shapes the future of care practices but also ensures that ethical AI implementation leads to a more compassionate and efficient care environment for the elderly and vulnerable.

Chapter 9: Conclusion: A Call to Action

The Ethical Imperative of AI in Care

The integration of artificial intelligence in residential care settings is not just a technological advancement; it represents an ethical imperative that must be embraced by private care home owners, NHS providers, and all stakeholders involved in elderly care. The historical focus on profit maximization in private care homes has often led to a neglect of quality care and inadequate staff training. As we move toward a future where generative AI can enhance the well-being of vulnerable populations, it is crucial to prioritize ethical considerations. This shift requires a commitment to using AI tools not only to improve efficiency but also to elevate the standards of care provided to residents.

Ethical AI practices can transform care home environments by ensuring that technology is used responsibly and effectively. Implementing AI systems that prioritize the needs and preferences of residents can lead to improved outcomes in their daily lives. For example, AI can assist in creating personalized care plans that take into account individual health conditions, preferences, and past experiences. By placing the resident at the center of care, these technologies can help foster a more compassionate and supportive atmosphere, countering the impersonal nature that can sometimes characterize care facilities.

Moreover, the potential for AI to reduce operational costs while enhancing care quality cannot be overstated. Through efficient resource management, AI tools can streamline administrative tasks, allowing staff to focus more on direct interactions with residents. This not only improves the quality of care provided but also mitigates the need for excessive staff cuts that often accompany a profit-driven model. With AI's ability to analyze data and predict care needs, facilities can allocate resources more effectively, ensuring that every resident receives the attention they deserve without compromising financial viability.

AI-assisted recreational activities also play a crucial role in enhancing the quality of life for elderly residents. By leveraging generative AI, care homes can develop tailored recreational programs that align with the interests and abilities of each individual. This customization not only fosters engagement but also promotes mental and emotional well-being. Activities designed through AI can adapt in real-time, responding to the residents' moods and preferences, ultimately creating a more dynamic and enjoyable living environment.

Finally, implementing AI in care homes provides data-driven insights that can significantly influence policy and practice improvements. By analyzing trends and outcomes, care facilities can identify areas requiring attention, adapt their strategies, and benchmark their performance against industry standards. This commitment to continuous improvement ensures that care homes are not only compliant with regulations but also proactive in enhancing resident care. As we embrace AI technologies in the care sector, we must remain steadfast in our ethical obligations to prioritize the dignity and autonomy of every individual, ensuring that the future of care is built on a foundation of compassion and respect.

Engaging Stakeholders for Sustainable Change

Engaging stakeholders for sustainable change in the context of care homes requires a collaborative approach that emphasizes shared goals and mutual benefits. Private care home owners, NHS representatives, healthcare professionals, and elderly care advocates must come together to foster an environment where ethical AI practices can thrive. This collaboration is essential not only for integrating generative AI solutions but also for ensuring that these technologies are aligned with the best interests of the elderly and vulnerable populations. By actively involving all stakeholders in the decision-making processes, care homes can create a framework that prioritizes quality care over profit margins.

One of the primary challenges faced by care homes is the historical focus on cost-cutting measures that often compromise the quality of care provided. By engaging stakeholders in discussions about the ethical implementation of AI, care homes can pivot away from this detrimental model. Stakeholders can collectively explore innovative solutions that utilize AI to enhance care without sacrificing staff training or resident well-being. This includes developing training programs for existing staff to better understand and operate AI tools, thus ensuring that technology complements rather than replaces human interaction.

Moreover, the integration of generative AI can lead to significant cost savings through efficient resource management. By involving stakeholders in the evaluation of AI technologies, care homes can identify tools that streamline operations, reduce waste, and optimize staffing levels. This collaborative approach enables the sharing of best practices and lessons learned, ultimately leading to more sustainable financial models. Stakeholders can work together to create a standardized framework for assessing the effectiveness of AI systems, ensuring that investments yield measurable improvements in care quality and operational efficiency.

AI-assisted recreational activities tailored to individual preferences are another area where stakeholder engagement is crucial. By gathering input from residents, families, and care staff, care homes can design programs that enhance the quality of life for elderly residents. Stakeholders can use data-driven insights to identify the most effective recreational activities, addressing not just physical well-being but also social and emotional health. This participatory approach fosters a sense of community and belonging, which is essential for the mental health of residents.

Finally, data-driven insights gained from stakeholder engagement can inform care home policies and practices to ensure they are both effective and ethical. By analyzing data on resident outcomes, stakeholder feedback, and AI performance metrics, care homes can adapt their strategies to better meet the needs of their residents. This ongoing dialogue between stakeholders creates a culture of transparency and accountability, where the primary focus remains on enhancing the quality of care. As care homes move toward a more sustainable future, the active engagement of all stakeholders will be key to navigating the complexities of ethical AI implementation.

Vision for the Future of Care in Residential Facilities

The vision for the future of care in residential facilities centers on integrating ethical AI practices that prioritize the well-being of elderly and vulnerable residents. This future aims to transcend the profit-driven motives that have historically characterized some private care homes, focusing instead on delivering high-quality care and employing well-trained staff. By embracing generative artificial intelligence, care homes can enhance their service offerings, ensuring that each resident receives personalized attention and support that meets their unique needs. This shift not only improves the quality of care but also fosters a more compassionate environment where residents feel valued and respected.

Implementing ethical AI in care home environments necessitates a commitment to transparency and accountability. Care home owners and operators must prioritize hiring trained professionals who can effectively utilize AI tools to augment their caregiving capabilities. This approach encourages a culture of continuous learning and adaptation, where staff are equipped to understand and implement AI-driven solutions that enhance resident care. As AI technologies advance, they can provide real-time insights into individual health statuses, allowing caregivers to respond proactively to changes in residents' conditions and ensuring that care is both timely and appropriate.

Reducing care costs through efficient AI resource management is another critical aspect of the future vision. By leveraging data analytics and AI-driven decision-making, care homes can optimize staffing levels, manage inventory more effectively, and streamline administrative processes. This not only reduces operational expenses but also allows for reinvestment in staff training and development. Ultimately, the goal is to create a sustainable financial model that supports high-quality care without compromising on the resources available to residents and staff alike.

AI-assisted recreational activities tailored to individual preferences will revolutionize how residents engage with their environment and each other. By utilizing generative AI to create personalized activity plans based on residents' interests and abilities, care homes can promote greater social interaction and mental stimulation. Such initiatives not only enhance the quality of life for residents but also contribute to a sense of community within the facility. This personalized approach to leisure activities fosters a more holistic view of care, where emotional and psychological well-being are prioritized alongside physical health.

Finally, data-driven insights will play a pivotal role in shaping care home policies and practices in the future. By harnessing AI to analyze trends in resident care, facilities can identify areas for improvement, develop targeted interventions, and implement evidence-based practices that enhance overall care quality. This proactive stance allows care homes to be agile and responsive to the evolving needs of their residents, ensuring that policies are not only effective but also aligned with the best practices in ethical care. Together, these elements form a comprehensive vision for the future of care in residential facilities, where technology and compassion coexist to create a nurturing environment for all.